The New Prepper's survival natural medicine

Learn How to Use Natural Medicine to Survive and Thrive in an Emergency

DALE FISHER

TABLE OF CONTENTS

Introduction

In an era marked by uncertainty and unpredictability, the need for self-sufficiency and resilience has never been more apparent. The fusion of natural medicine and emergency preparedness offers a potent antidote to the vulnerabilities of modern life. In this introduction, we delve into the inherent benefits of natural medicine, underscore the critical importance of emergency preparedness, and outline the invaluable knowledge that awaits within the pages of this book.

The Benefits of Natural Medicine

Natural medicine, rooted in centuries-old wisdom and practices, harnesses the innate healing powers of nature to promote holistic well-being. Unlike conventional pharmaceuticals, which often come laden with side effects and synthetic compounds, natural remedies offer gentler, yet effective alternatives.

From herbal teas to essential oils, these remedies work in harmony with the body's natural processes, stimulating its innate ability to heal itself.

Moreover, natural medicine champions a preventative approach to health, empowering individuals to cultivate resilience and vitality from within. By bolstering the body's immune system and addressing underlying imbalances, natural remedies not only alleviate symptoms but also fortify the body's defenses against future ailments. This proactive stance towards health not only enhances physical vitality but also fosters a profound sense of empowerment and self-reliance.

The Importance of Emergency Preparedness

In an increasingly volatile world, characterized by natural disasters, geopolitical unrest, and unforeseen crises, the importance of emergency preparedness cannot be overstated. Emergencies can strike suddenly and without warning, leaving individuals and communities vulnerable to chaos and devastation. However, by adopting a proactive approach to preparedness, individuals can mitigate risks, enhance resilience, and safeguard the well-being of themselves and their loved ones.

Emergency preparedness encompasses a multifaceted approach, encompassing everything from stockpiling essential supplies to developing evacuation plans and acquiring crucial life-saving skills. By cultivating a mindset of readiness and resilience, individuals can navigate emergencies with greater confidence and efficacy, minimizing the impact of disasters and facilitating swift recovery.

What Readers Can Expect to Learn

Within the pages of this book, readers will embark on a transformative journey towards self-sufficiency, empowerment, and resilience. Drawing upon the timeless wisdom of natural medicine and the pragmatic principles of emergency preparedness, readers will gain invaluable insights, skills, and strategies to navigate emergencies with confidence and competence.

Readers can expect to learn a comprehensive array of natural remedies for common ailments and injuries, ranging from herbal remedies to essential oils and homeopathic treatments. Each remedy will be accompanied by detailed descriptions and step-by-step instructions, empowering readers to harness the healing powers of nature effectively.

Furthermore, readers will discover specialized natural remedies tailored to specific emergency situations, such as natural disasters, power outages, and food shortages. From building robust emergency kits to cultivating emergency communication plans, readers will acquire practical knowledge and actionable strategies to weather crises with resilience and resourcefulness.

Lastly, readers will find a curated list of resources, including websites, books, and organizations, offering further support and information on natural medicine and emergency preparedness. This invaluable compilation serves as a roadmap for continued learning and exploration, enabling readers to deepen their understanding and expand their preparedness toolkit.

In essence, this book serves as a comprehensive guidebook for individuals seeking to embrace the transformative power of natural medicine and cultivate resilience in the face of adversity. Through its clear, concise, and authoritative approach, it empowers readers to not only survive but thrive in emergencies, embodying the ethos of self-reliance, empowerment, and preparedness.

Section 1: Natural Remedies for Common Ailments and Injuries

In times of emergency, access to conventional medical care may be limited or unavailable. As such, knowing how to harness the healing power of nature becomes paramount. In this section, we delve into a comprehensive array of natural remedies for common ailments and injuries, equipping readers with the knowledge and skills to address health challenges effectively and confidently.

Chapter 1: Herbal Remedies

Herbal remedies, derived from various plant parts such as leaves, roots, flowers, and seeds, have been utilized for centuries by cultures worldwide for their medicinal properties. Harnessing the therapeutic compounds found in plants, herbal remedies offer gentle yet potent solutions for a myriad of health concerns. In this chapter, we explore the diverse world of herbal medicine, highlighting key remedies and their applications.

Common Herbal Remedies:

Echinacea (Echinacea purpurea): Widely revered for its immune-boosting properties, echinacea is commonly used to prevent and treat upper respiratory infections, such as the common cold and flu. Its anti-inflammatory and antiviral effects help shorten the duration and severity of symptoms, making it a valuable addition to any prepper's medicine cabinet.

Ginger (Zingiber officinale): A staple in traditional medicine, ginger boasts a myriad of health benefits, including anti-nausea, anti-inflammatory, and digestive support properties. Whether consumed as a tea, chewed raw, or applied topically, ginger can alleviate nausea, soothe sore muscles, and promote overall well-being, making it an indispensable remedy in times of distress.

Arnica (Arnica montana): Recognized for its analgesic and anti-inflammatory properties, arnica is commonly used topically to relieve pain and inflammation associated with bruises, sprains, and muscle soreness. Its natural healing compounds penetrate deep into the skin, reducing swelling and promoting tissue repair, facilitating faster recovery from injuries.

Application and Dosage:

When utilizing herbal remedies, proper application and dosage are essential for optimal efficacy and safety. While some herbs can be consumed orally as teas, tinctures, or capsules, others are best used topically as poultices, compresses, or infused oils. It's crucial to follow recommended dosage guidelines and consult with a healthcare professional, especially when using potent herbs or combining multiple remedies.

Storage and Preparation:

To maintain the potency and shelf-life of herbal remedies, proper storage and preparation are paramount. Store dried herbs in airtight containers away from direct sunlight and moisture to prevent degradation. When preparing herbal preparations, such as teas or tinctures, use high-quality herbs and follow precise instructions to ensure optimal extraction of medicinal compounds.

Chapter 2: Essential Oils and Their Uses

Essential oils, aromatic compounds extracted from plants through steam distillation or cold pressing, are prized for their potent therapeutic properties. From soothing sore muscles to alleviating stress and promoting relaxation, essential oils offer a myriad of health benefits for both body and mind. In this chapter, we explore the versatile uses of essential oils and their applications in emergency situations.

Common Essential Oils:

Lavender (Lavandula angustifolia):
Renowned for its calming and sedative properties, lavender essential oil is a versatile remedy for stress, anxiety, and insomnia. Its gentle aroma promotes relaxation, soothes the nervous system, and aids in restful sleep, making it an invaluable ally during times of heightened tension and uncertainty.

Tea Tree (Melaleuca alternifolia): With its powerful antimicrobial and antiseptic properties, tea tree essential oil is a potent remedy for skin infections, cuts, and wounds. Its natural cleansing action helps prevent infection and promote rapid healing, making it an essential addition to first aid kits and emergency preparedness supplies.

Peppermint (Mentha piperita): Known for its cooling and invigorating effects, peppermint essential oil is a go-to remedy for headaches, nausea, and digestive discomfort. Its analgesic properties provide quick relief from tension headaches, while its anti-nausea effects alleviate symptoms of motion sickness and indigestion, offering much-needed comfort during emergencies.

Application Methods:

Essential oils can be applied topically, inhaled, or ingested, depending on the desired effect and the oil's specific properties. When using essential oils topically, dilute them with a carrier oil, such as coconut or almond oil, to prevent skin irritation. Inhalation methods, such as diffusing or steam inhalation, allow for quick absorption of aromatic compounds, promoting respiratory health and emotional well-being.

Safety Considerations:

While essential oils offer numerous health benefits, it's essential to use them safely and responsibly. Some oils may cause skin irritation or allergic reactions, especially when used undiluted or in high concentrations. Additionally, certain oils may be contraindicated for pregnant women, children, or individuals with specific medical conditions. Always perform a patch test and consult with a qualified aromatherapist or healthcare professional before using essential oils, particularly in emergency situations.

Chapter 3: Homeopathic Treatments

Homeopathy, a system of alternative medicine based on the principle of "like cures like," utilizes highly diluted remedies to stimulate the body's innate healing mechanisms. By addressing the underlying root cause of symptoms, homeopathic treatments offer gentle yet effective solutions for a wide range of health conditions. In this chapter, we explore the principles of homeopathy and its applications in emergency care.

Principles of Homeopathy:

Homeopathy operates on the principle of "vital force," the innate energy that governs the body's ability to heal itself. Remedies are selected based on the principle of "similarity," wherein a substance that produces symptoms in a healthy individual is used to treat similar symptoms in a sick individual. These remedies are prepared through a process of potentization, wherein they are diluted and succussed (vigorously shaken) to enhance their therapeutic potency while minimizing toxicity.

Common Homeopathic Remedies:

Arnica montana: A cornerstone remedy in homeopathy, arnica is renowned for its ability to alleviate trauma, bruising, and shock. Whether used orally or topically, arnica promotes rapid healing and reduces inflammation, making it an indispensable remedy for injuries, falls, and accidents.

Aconitum napellus: Known as the "king of acute remedies," aconite is indicated for sudden onset conditions, such as fevers, colds, and panic attacks. Its calming and sedative effects help alleviate symptoms of anxiety, restlessness, and fear, restoring balance and equilibrium to the body and mind.

Apis mellifica: Derived from the honeybee, apis is a potent remedy for allergic reactions, insect bites, and inflammatory conditions. Its anti-inflammatory and antihistaminic properties soothe itching, swelling, and redness, providing rapid relief from allergic symptoms and insect stings.

Administration and Dosage:

Homeopathic remedies are typically administered in highly diluted form, either in pellet, liquid, or topical form. Depending on the severity and nature of symptoms, remedies may be taken orally, applied topically, or inhaled as needed. Dosage and potency selection vary depending on individual sensitivity and response, with lower potencies often recommended for acute conditions and higher potencies for chronic ailments.

Integration with Conventional Medicine:

While homeopathy is often utilized as a standalone therapy, it can also complement conventional medical treatments, offering a holistic approach to health and healing.

Integrating homeopathic remedies with conventional medicine can enhance treatment outcomes, minimize side effects, and promote overall well-being. However, it's essential to consult with a qualified homeopath or healthcare professional before combining therapies to ensure compatibility and safety.

Emergency Applications:

In emergency situations, homeopathic remedies offer rapid relief from a wide range of acute symptoms and conditions. Whether addressing injuries, infections, or emotional trauma, homeopathy provides gentle yet effective solutions for restoring balance and promoting healing. By supporting the body's innate healing mechanisms, homeopathic treatments can help individuals navigate emergencies with resilience and resourcefulness, mitigating the impact of injuries and promoting swift recovery.

Case Examples:

Injury Relief: In cases of trauma, such as falls or accidents, arnica is often the remedy of choice for reducing pain, swelling, and bruising. Administered orally or applied topically as a cream or gel, arnica promotes rapid healing and minimizes the severity of injuries, allowing individuals to resume normal activities more quickly.

Allergic Reactions: In instances of allergic reactions, such as insect stings or food allergies, apis mellifica can provide rapid relief from itching, swelling, and redness. Taken orally or applied topically as a cream or ointment, apis helps counteract the inflammatory response and restore balance to the immune system, alleviating discomfort and promoting recovery.

Acute Illness: In cases of sudden onset illnesses, such as fevers, colds, or flu-like symptoms, aconitum napellus can help mitigate symptoms of anxiety, restlessness, and fear. Administered orally in pellet form or diluted in water, aconite supports the body's natural defenses and helps restore equilibrium, facilitating a swift resolution of symptoms.

Conclusion:

Incorporating herbal remedies, essential oils, and homeopathic treatments into your emergency preparedness toolkit empowers you to address common ailments and injuries effectively and confidently. By harnessing the healing power of nature, you can enhance resilience, promote well-being, and navigate emergencies with grace and resilience. Whether you're preparing for natural disasters, power outages, or unexpected crises, these natural remedies offer invaluable support and guidance for thriving in challenging times. As you embark on your journey towards self-sufficiency and preparedness, may these remedies serve as trusted allies in your quest for health, vitality, and peace of mind.

Section 2: Natural Remedies for Specific Emergency Situations

In times of crisis, such as natural disasters, power outages, and food shortages, access to conventional medical care and resources may become severely limited. However, by harnessing the healing power of nature and adopting a proactive approach to preparedness, individuals can navigate these challenges with resilience and resourcefulness. In this section, we explore a range of natural remedies and strategies tailored to specific emergency situations, empowering readers to thrive in the face of adversity.

Chapter 4: Preparing for Natural Disasters

Natural disasters, such as hurricanes, earthquakes, wildfires, and floods, pose significant threats to life, property, and infrastructure. In the event of a disaster, access to medical care and essential resources may be compromised, necessitating a proactive approach to preparedness. In this chapter, we discuss key strategies for preparing for natural disasters and utilizing natural remedies to address common health concerns in emergency situations.

Emergency Preparedness:

Developing a Comprehensive Emergency Plan: Begin by creating a detailed emergency plan that includes evacuation routes, communication protocols, and designated meeting points for family members. Consider the specific hazards and risks in your region and tailor your plan accordingly to ensure maximum preparedness.

Building an Emergency Supply Kit: Assemble a well-stocked emergency supply kit that includes essential items such as water, non-perishable food, first aid supplies, flashlights, batteries, and personal hygiene products. Consider incorporating natural remedies such as herbal teas, essential oils, and homeopathic treatments to address common health concerns during emergencies.

Securing Your Home and Property: Take proactive measures to secure your home and property against potential damage from natural disasters. Trim trees and bushes, reinforce windows and doors, and secure loose objects that could become projectiles in high winds. Install smoke detectors and carbon monoxide alarms to ensure early detection of hazards.

Natural Remedies for Common Health Concerns:

Stress and Anxiety: Natural remedies such as lavender essential oil, chamomile tea, and rescue remedy (a combination of flower essences) can help alleviate stress and anxiety during times of crisis. Practice relaxation techniques such as deep breathing, meditation, and yoga to promote emotional well-being and resilience.

Wound Care: Injuries are common during natural disasters, so it's essential to have supplies on hand for wound care. Cleanse wounds with diluted antiseptic solutions such as tea tree oil or calendula tincture, and apply natural wound-healing ointments such as comfrey or plantain salve to promote tissue repair and prevent infection.

Respiratory Health: Poor air quality due to smoke, dust, or pollutants can exacerbate respiratory conditions such as asthma and allergies. Use natural remedies such as eucalyptus essential oil or peppermint steam inhalations to clear congestion and soothe irritated airways. Consider wearing a mask or respirator when venturing outdoors in hazardous conditions.

Chapter 5: Coping with Power Outages

Power outages can occur unexpectedly due to severe weather, equipment failure, or grid disruptions, leaving individuals without access to electricity for extended periods. In addition to the inconvenience of being without lights and appliances, power outages can also pose health and safety risks. In this chapter, we explore natural remedies and strategies for coping with power outages and maintaining health and well-being in adverse conditions.

Emergency Preparedness:

Stockpiling Emergency Supplies: Prepare for power outages by stocking up on essential supplies such as bottled water, non-perishable food, batteries, flashlights, and portable chargers for electronic devices. Consider investing in alternative energy sources such as solar panels or portable generators to provide backup power during emergencies.

Ensuring Food Safety: During power outages, the safety of perishable foods such as meat, dairy, and leftovers may be compromised. Keep refrigerators and freezers closed as much as possible to maintain cold temperatures, and use perishable items first before turning to non-perishable alternatives. Monitor food temperatures with a digital thermometer and discard any items that have been exposed to unsafe temperatures for an extended period.

Maintaining Indoor Comfort: Without electricity for heating or cooling, indoor temperatures can become uncomfortable and potentially dangerous. Stay warm during cold weather by layering clothing, using blankets, and huddling together for body heat. In hot weather, seek shelter in cool, shaded areas, and stay hydrated to prevent heat-related illnesses such as heat exhaustion and heatstroke.

Natural Remedies for Common Health Concerns:

Heat-related Illnesses: During power outages, the risk of heat-related illnesses such as heat exhaustion and heatstroke increases, especially in hot and humid climates. Stay cool by taking frequent cool showers or baths, using fans or battery-operated portable fans, and applying cool compresses to the neck and wrists. Drink plenty of water to stay hydrated and avoid caffeinated or alcoholic beverages, which can contribute to dehydration.

Food Poisoning: Without refrigeration, perishable foods can spoil quickly, increasing the risk of foodborne illness. Practice food safety measures such as keeping raw and cooked foods separate, cooking foods to the appropriate temperature, and refrigerating leftovers promptly. If food poisoning occurs, stay hydrated with clear fluids and consider natural remedies such as activated charcoal or ginger tea to alleviate symptoms of nausea and vomiting.

Sleep Disturbances: Disrupted sleep patterns due to discomfort or anxiety can exacerbate stress and fatigue during power outages. Create a comfortable sleep environment by using breathable bedding, keeping rooms well-ventilated, and reducing noise and light disturbances. Practice relaxation techniques such as deep breathing or guided imagery to promote restful sleep and alleviate nighttime anxiety.

Chapter 6: Surviving Food Shortages

Food shortages can occur due to various factors such as crop failures, transportation disruptions, or supply chain interruptions, leaving individuals without access to an adequate food supply. In emergency situations, it's essential to have a plan in place for managing food shortages and ensuring nutritional adequacy. In this chapter, we explore natural remedies and strategies for surviving food shortages and maintaining health and well-being during times of scarcity.

Emergency Preparedness:

Building a Sustainable Food Supply: Prepare for food shortages by building a sustainable food supply that includes non-perishable staples such as grains, legumes, canned goods, and dried fruits and vegetables. Consider growing your own food in a garden or container garden, or participating in community-supported agriculture (CSA) programs to access fresh, locally grown produce.

Preserving Food: Extend the shelf life of perishable foods by preserving them through methods such as canning, pickling, drying, or fermenting. Invest in home food preservation equipment such as pressure canners, dehydrators, or fermentation crocks to process and store surplus produce for long-term use.

Exploring Alternative Food Sources: In times of scarcity, consider exploring alternative food sources such as foraging for wild edible plants, fishing, hunting, or raising backyard chickens or rabbits for meat and eggs. Learn to identify edible wild plants and mushrooms in your area, and practice ethical and sustainable harvesting practices to minimize environmental impact.

Natural Remedies for Nutritional Support:

During food shortages, it may be challenging to obtain an adequate intake of essential nutrients such as vitamins, minerals, and protein. Consider supplementing your diet with natural sources of nutrients such as spirulina, chlorella, or nutritional yeast, which are rich in vitamins, minerals, and protein. These supplements can help fill nutritional gaps and support overall health and well-being during times of scarcity.

Maximizing Nutrient Density: Make the most of limited food resources by prioritizing nutrient-dense foods that provide essential vitamins, minerals, and antioxidants. Focus on incorporating foods such as leafy greens, cruciferous vegetables, berries, nuts, seeds, and whole grains into your diet to optimize nutritional intake and support immune function.

Creating Balanced Meals: Despite food shortages, strive to create balanced meals that provide a variety of nutrients and macronutrients to meet your body's needs. Aim to include a combination of carbohydrates, protein, healthy fats, and fiber in each meal to promote satiety, energy, and overall health. Get creative with meal planning and preparation, using versatile ingredients and simple cooking techniques to maximize flavor and nutrition.

Emergency Nutrition Strategies:

Rationing Food Supplies: During food shortages, it's essential to ration food supplies wisely to ensure adequate nutrition for yourself and your family. Prioritize high-calorie, nutrient-dense foods such as grains, legumes, nuts, and dried fruits, and allocate portions based on energy needs and nutritional requirements. Avoid overeating or wasting food, and practice portion control to make supplies last longer.

Prioritizing Water Intake: In addition to food shortages, access to clean, potable water may also be limited during emergencies. Stay hydrated by prioritizing water intake and conserving water resources whenever possible. Consider investing in water purification methods such as portable water filters, purification tablets, or boiling water to ensure safe drinking water for you and your family.

Community Support and Collaboration: In times of crisis, community support and collaboration are essential for overcoming food shortages and ensuring the well-being of all members. Form alliances with neighbors, friends, and local organizations to share resources, pool collective skills and knowledge, and support one another through challenging times. Establish community gardens, food cooperatives, or meal-sharing programs to promote resilience and mutual aid within your community.

Natural Remedies for Health Maintenance:

Immune Support: Boost your immune system and protect against illness by incorporating immune-supportive herbs and supplements into your daily routine. Consider using natural remedies such as elderberry syrup, astragalus root, and medicinal mushrooms (e.g., reishi, shiitake, maitake) to enhance immune function and support overall health during times of stress and scarcity.

Stress Management: Maintain emotional well-being and resilience during food shortages by implementing stress management techniques such as mindfulness, meditation, and relaxation exercises. Practice self-care activities that promote relaxation and reduce anxiety, such as spending time in nature, engaging in creative pursuits, or connecting with loved ones.

Physical Activity: Stay active and maintain physical fitness during food shortages by incorporating regular exercise into your daily routine. Engage in activities such as walking, jogging, yoga, or bodyweight exercises that require minimal equipment and can be performed indoors or outdoors. Physical activity not only supports overall health and well-being but also helps alleviate stress and promote mental clarity during challenging times.

In conclusion, preparing for and navigating specific emergency situations such as natural disasters, power outages, and food shortages require a proactive approach and a comprehensive toolkit of natural remedies and strategies. By incorporating these remedies into your emergency preparedness plan, you can enhance resilience, promote well-being, and thrive in the face of adversity. Whether you're stocking up on herbal remedies for wound care, using essential oils to alleviate stress and anxiety, or exploring alternative food sources for nutritional support, these natural solutions offer invaluable support for surviving and thriving in challenging times. As you embark on your journey towards self-sufficiency and preparedness, may these remedies serve as trusted allies in your quest for health, vitality, and peace of mind.

Section 3: Resources for Further Information

In the quest for self-sufficiency and resilience, knowledge is key. In this section, we provide a curated list of resources to deepen your understanding of natural medicine, emergency preparedness, and community support. From authoritative websites and informative books to reputable organizations, these resources offer invaluable guidance and information to empower you on your journey towards survival and thriving in emergencies.

Chapter 7: Websites for Natural Medicine Resources

The internet is a treasure trove of information, providing access to a wealth of resources on natural medicine, herbal remedies, and holistic health practices. However, not all websites are created equal, and it's essential to discern reliable sources from misinformation. In this chapter, we highlight reputable websites that offer credible information and resources on natural medicine and complementary therapies.

National Center for Complementary and Integrative Health (NCCIH): As part of the National Institutes of Health (NIH), the NCCIH is a leading authority on complementary and alternative medicine. Their website offers evidence-based information on herbs, supplements, and mind-body practices, as well as research updates and clinical trials.

American Herbalists Guild (AHG): The AHG is a professional organization dedicated to promoting the practice of herbalism and supporting herbal practitioners. Their website features educational resources, articles, and a directory of qualified herbalists, making it a valuable resource for those interested in herbal medicine.

Herbal Academy: The Herbal Academy is an online platform offering courses, articles, and resources on herbalism and natural health. Their website provides comprehensive information on herbal remedies, plant identification, and herbal preparations, catering to both beginners and experienced herbalists.

PubMed: Operated by the National Library of Medicine, PubMed is a database of biomedical literature containing millions of articles on health-related topics. While primarily geared towards healthcare professionals, PubMed is a valuable resource for accessing scientific research on herbs, supplements, and alternative therapies.

The Herb Society of America (HSA): The HSA is a nonprofit organization dedicated to promoting the knowledge, use, and appreciation of herbs. Their website offers educational materials, publications, and resources on herb gardening, culinary herbs, and medicinal plants, serving as a valuable resource for herb enthusiasts and gardeners.

Chapter 8: Books on Emergency Preparedness

In times of crisis, having reliable reference materials at your disposal can make all the difference. Books on emergency preparedness offer practical guidance, actionable strategies, and expert advice for navigating a wide range of emergency scenarios. In this chapter, we recommend essential books that cover various aspects of emergency preparedness, from survival skills to disaster planning.

"The SAS Survival Handbook" by John "Lofty" Wiseman: Widely regarded as a classic in the field of survival literature, "The SAS Survival Handbook" provides comprehensive guidance on wilderness survival, emergency first aid, shelter building, and navigation. With detailed illustrations and practical tips, this book is an indispensable resource for anyone seeking to develop essential survival skills.

"Emergency Food Storage & Survival Handbook" by Peggy Layton: In this practical guide, Peggy Layton offers expert advice on stockpiling food, water, and supplies for emergencies. From pantry staples to long-term food storage solutions, this book provides step-by-step instructions and budget-friendly tips for building a robust emergency food supply.

"The Prepper's Blueprint" by Tess Pennington: "The Prepper's Blueprint" offers a comprehensive guide to preparedness planning, covering everything from risk assessment and emergency communication to self-defense and community resilience. With actionable checklists and real-life case studies, this book equips readers with the knowledge and skills needed to thrive in any emergency situation.

"Where There Is No Doctor" by David Werner: Written for healthcare workers in resource-limited settings, "Where There Is No Doctor" provides practical information on basic healthcare, disease prevention, and medical treatment. With emphasis on low-cost, accessible solutions, this book offers invaluable insights into providing medical care in austere environments.

"Build the Perfect Bug Out Bag" by Creek Stewart: In "Build the Perfect Bug Out Bag," Creek Stewart offers expert guidance on assembling a comprehensive emergency kit for evacuation scenarios. From essential gear and tools to survival tactics and navigation skills, this book provides practical advice for building and maintaining a bug out bag for emergencies.

Chapter 9: Organizations Providing Support and Information

In times of crisis, community support and collaboration are essential for resilience and recovery. Fortunately, there are numerous organizations dedicated to providing support, information, and resources to individuals and communities in need. In this chapter, we highlight reputable organizations that offer assistance, guidance, and solidarity in times of emergencies.

American Red Cross: As a leading humanitarian organization, the American Red Cross provides disaster relief, emergency preparedness education, and community support services across the United States. From sheltering and feeding to first aid training and emotional support, the Red Cross offers a range of services to help individuals and communities prepare for, respond to, and recover from disasters.

Federal Emergency Management Agency (FEMA): FEMA is the federal agency responsible for coordinating disaster response and recovery efforts in the United States. Their website offers resources on emergency preparedness, disaster planning, and recovery assistance, including information on how to access federal aid and assistance programs in the event of a disaster.

Volunteer Organizations Active in Disaster (VOAD): VOAD is a national network of nonprofit organizations dedicated to providing disaster relief and recovery services. With chapters in every state, VOAD members collaborate to deliver essential services such as sheltering, feeding, and emotional support to disaster-affected communities.

Community Emergency Response Teams (CERT): CERT is a community-based program that trains volunteers to assist emergency responders in disaster situations. CERT members receive training in basic disaster response skills, such as first aid, fire safety, search and rescue, and disaster psychology, enabling them to support their communities during emergencies.

Local Health Departments: Local health departments play a crucial role in emergency preparedness and response, providing public health services, medical care, and disease surveillance in their communities. Contact your local health department for information on emergency preparedness resources, vaccination clinics, and community health initiatives in your area.

In conclusion, access to reliable information and support is essential for preparing for and navigating emergencies effectively. Whether seeking guidance on natural medicine, emergency preparedness, or community support services, these resources offer valuable insights, expertise, and assistance to empower individuals and communities in times of need. By leveraging these resources and building collaborative networks, we can strengthen our resilience, promote well-being, and thrive in the face of adversity.

Glossary of Terms

1. **Natural Medicine:** Healing practices that utilize natural remedies, such as herbs, essential oils, and homeopathic treatments, to promote health and well-being.

2. **Emergency Preparedness:** The process of planning and preparing for potential emergencies or disasters, including natural disasters, power outages, and food shortages, to mitigate risks and ensure survival.

3. **Herbal Remedies:** Medicinal preparations made from plants, including leaves, roots, flowers, and seeds, used to treat or alleviate various health conditions.

4. **Essential Oils:** Concentrated aromatic compounds extracted from plants through steam distillation or cold pressing, used for their therapeutic properties in aromatherapy and natural medicine.

5. **Homeopathic Treatments:** A system of alternative medicine based on the principle of "like cures like," using highly diluted remedies to stimulate the body's self-healing mechanisms.

6. **Resilience:** The ability to adapt and recover from adversity, including the capacity to bounce back from emergencies or crises.

7. **Preparedness Kit:** A collection of essential supplies and resources assembled in advance to help individuals and families cope with emergencies, including food, water, first aid supplies, and communication devices.

8. **Sustainable Living:** A lifestyle focused on reducing environmental impact and promoting self-sufficiency through practices such as gardening, composting, and renewable energy usage.

9. **Community Resilience:** The collective ability of a community to respond to and recover

from emergencies or disasters, involving collaboration, resource-sharing, and mutual support among community members.

10. **Self-Sufficiency:** The ability to meet one's basic needs, such as food, water, and shelter, without relying on external assistance or infrastructure.

11. **Alternative Medicine:** Healing practices and therapies that fall outside the scope of conventional Western medicine, including natural medicine, acupuncture, and traditional Chinese medicine.

12. **Preparedness Planning:** The process of developing and implementing strategies to anticipate and mitigate risks, including creating emergency plans, stockpiling supplies, and practicing response protocols.

13. **Nutrient Density:** The concentration of essential nutrients, such as vitamins, minerals, and antioxidants, in a given food or dietary

pattern, reflecting its nutritional value per calorie.

14. **Emergency Response:** The organized efforts to address and mitigate the immediate consequences of an emergency or disaster, including rescue operations, medical care, and disaster relief efforts.

15. **First Aid:** Initial medical care and treatment provided to individuals experiencing illness or injury, typically administered by trained individuals or first responders until professional medical help arrives.

16. **Natural Disaster:** Severe or catastrophic events caused by natural phenomena, such as hurricanes, earthquakes, floods, wildfires, or tornadoes, resulting in widespread damage and disruption.

17. **Adaptability:** The capacity to adjust and respond effectively to changing circumstances or

environments, including unforeseen challenges or emergencies.

18. **Preparedness Education:** The dissemination of knowledge, skills, and resources to individuals and communities to enhance their readiness and resilience in the face of emergencies or disasters.

19. **Sustainability:** The practice of meeting present needs without compromising the ability of future generations to meet their own needs, encompassing environmental, social, and economic dimensions.

20. **Self-Care:** Practices and activities undertaken to promote physical, mental, and emotional well-being, including relaxation techniques, healthy eating, exercise, and stress management.

Index

A

E

F

H

S

Self-Care,

Self-Sufficiency,

Sustainability,

W

Websites for Natural Medicine Resources,